Getting Healthy

5 Permanent Lifestyle Changes That Help Achieve Your Fitness Goals

Ron Kness

No part of this book may be reproduced, stored in a retrieval system, or transmitted in any form or by any means, electronic, mechanical, photocopying, recording, scanning, or otherwise, without the prior written permission of the publisher, except for the inclusion of brief quotations in a review.

This book is for **personal use only**.

Published by:

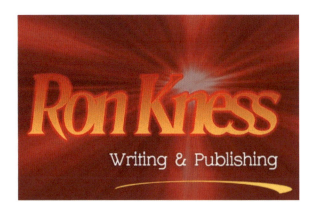

https://ronknesswriting.com

Ron Kness

Queen Creek, AZ

United States of America

For

Healthy Lifestyle Newsletter

https://healthylifestylenewsletter.com

ISBN: 9798747580428

Copyright © 2021 – Ron Kness – All Rights Reserved

Disclaimer

This publication is for informational purposes only and is not intended as medical advice. Medical advice should always be obtained from a qualified medical professional for any health conditions or symptoms associated with them.

Every possible effort has been made in preparing and researching this material. We make no warranties with respect to the accuracy, applicability of its contents or any omissions.

See your healthcare professional before starting any diet, health or exercise program!

Contents

Disclaimer 3

Keeping It Real – Don't Do Too Much Too Fast 7

Stop Making Excuses 9

Getting Back On Track – How To Pick Yourself Up After Falling Off Your Diet 11

How To Set Smart Weight Loss Goals 13

Set Yourself Up For Success – How To Stick To Your Weight Loss Goals 15

Lifestyle Changes 17

    #1 - Eat Less 17

        Portion Control 17

        Group Your Foods Correctly 18

        Drink Plenty Of Water 18

    #2 - Eat Better 19

        Less Sugar 19

        Less Carbs 19

        More Protein 19

        More Non-Starchy Veggies 20

        Healthy Fats 20

    #3 - Move More 20

    #4 - Choose Your Passion 21

    #5 - Get Support 21

Smart Apps To Help You Reach Your Weight Loss Goals 23

Tools To Help You Reach Your Weight Loss Goals 26

From Overweight to In Shape - 6 Smart Goal Setting Tips 28

Reaching Weight Loss Milestones - Don't Forget To Celebrate Your Success 31

About the Author 33

Life Happens – Don't Give Up On Your Health Goals

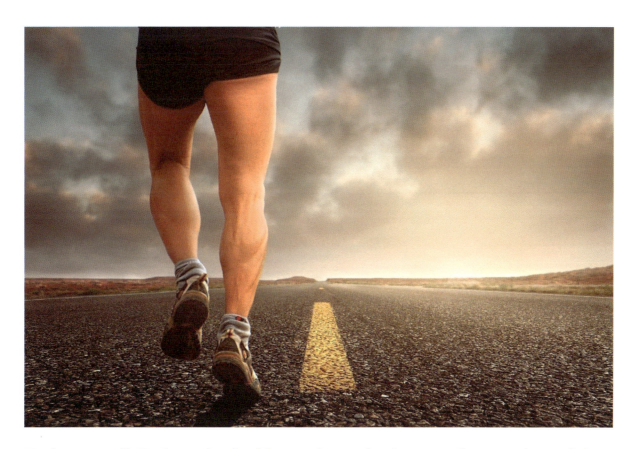

You're on a roll. You're eating healthy, you're getting into a workout routine and the pounds are starting to melt off. Then life happens. You get sick, your schedule changes, you're tempted by your favorite treat. The reason really doesn't matter. The truth is that you fell off the wagon and ate some unhealthy food and didn't make it to your weekly workout.

When stuff like that happens it's easy to give up. A day of eating junk can turn into a week and then a month. A few days spent without going for a walk, a run or a trip to the gym turn into weeks. Don't let that happen. When life happens – and it will – refuse to give up on your health goals.

The key is to get back into your routine as quickly as possible. Don't beat yourself up about it. Instead, make it a priority to jump right back in. Get back to your healthy eating habits and get your body moving as soon as possible. Even if it's just a little exercise here and there during a super busy time, make the effort to do what you can. Every little bit helps and every small step is a step in the right direction. 15 minutes at a time can make a big difference in the long run.

It helps to be prepared for potential pitfalls. For example, if you know things will get super busy at work and you won't have time to head out for a healthy lunch or to go on your daily walk, make some plans the day before.

Pack your lunch just in case you end up working through your lunch hour. At the very least you'll still have a healthy meal.

Do little things to help you keep on track. Things like walking around during phone calls, a 15-minute mini- workout or a walk before work. Try doing some simple stretches before bed. Little things like this will add up and help you relieve some of the stress you're under.

Keep some healthy snacks and plenty of water with you so you can make smart choices when hunger strikes. If time is precious and you just don't have the extra hour or two to head to the gym or go for a walk, do little mini workouts throughout your day. Do some stretches, a few push-ups or walk over to a colleague's desk instead of calling him.

Remember, every little bit counts and each step you take to a healthier you is a step in the right direction.

I hate to break it to you, but there is no easy way to get healthy, lose weight or get back into shape. It takes time and it takes dedication. Yes, it would be nice to have a magical pill or an easy button. That's the reason there's such a huge market for diet pills and weight loss gimmicks. But the hard truth is that they just don't work.

What works is making lifestyle changes and sticking to them. That's what this short report is all about. I'm not promising that it will be easy as pie or that you'll lose 50 pounds overnight. What I can promise is some helpful information that will allow you to make those lifestyle changes. I'll show you how to create good habits that will help you reach your goals. After that it's up to you to implement them and finally get healthy – for life.

Keeping It Real – Don't Do Too Much Too Fast

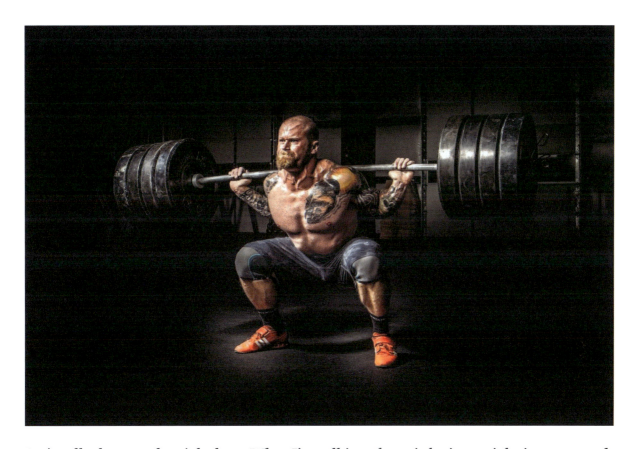

Let's talk about real weight loss. What I'm talking about is losing weight in a way and at a rate that's sustainable. Yes, you can go on one of those miracle liquid diets for 48 hours and lose a few pounds. But it isn't something you'd want to (or should) be sticking with for the long run. Plus chances are that as soon as you go back to eating normally you'll get the weight right back.

Instead I'd like to make a case for slow and steady weight loss. You didn't put those 30 extra pounds on overnight. Don't expect to take them off in a matter of weeks. Instead, aim to lose half a pound to a pound per week. Believe me, it'll still be a challenge most weeks.

The key to slow and steady weight loss is lifestyle changes. The changes you make to your lifestyle today should become habits that will stick with you forever.

Drink more water, cut out high calorie drinks like soda and fruit juices. Cut back on sugar and refined carbs as much as possible. Stick with low sugar fruits, lots of non-starchy veggies and protein. Don't forget to add a few healthy fats. Yes, they are high in calories, but they'll also keep you full longer.

Make it a habit to go for a 30-minute walk after dinner in the evening. Or start a yoga class. Try to move around more all throughout your day.

Get up and walk around while you're talking on the phone. Go play with the kids in the yard or ride a bike. Keep in mind that you can move in 15-minute spurts to meet your daily goals.

Small lifestyle changes will start to add up and you'll see some slow and steady weight loss. And there's another important reason why you want to keep it real and not try to do too much too fast. The end goal is to keep the weight off. And that will be easier with if you do it slowly by changing the way you eat, the way you move and your whole outlook on life. Set yourself up for success by setting small weight loss goals and working toward them.

Yes it takes some patience, but it will be well worth it in the end. Because the end goal is a healthier, more active version of you. Someone that can run around with the kids at the park. Someone that's setting a great example for her loved ones. And yes, someone that fits in that pretty new dress.

Stop Making Excuses

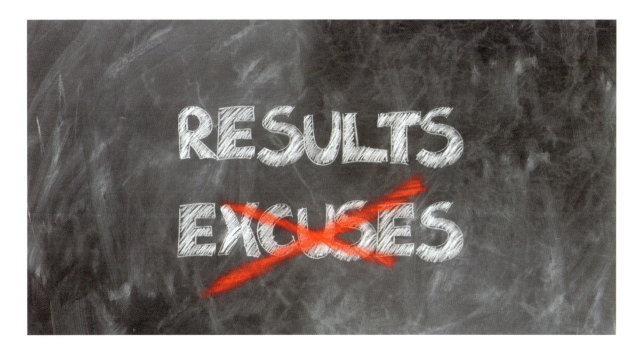

If you want to get down to a healthy weight, you have to stop making excuses. You know what I'm talking about. It's that little voice in the back of your head that tells you that you deserve to eat that doughnut because you've had a rough morning. Or the one that tells you that it's too cold to go out for your nightly walk. We all have that little voice in our head. We also all have a choice each time that voice speaks up. We can listen to it, or we can choose to ignore it.

Ignoring that little voice and not making excuses isn't easy, particularly in the beginning. But here's the good news. As you start to ignore it more and more often and go work out, or say no to the high-sugar, high-calorie treat, the softer that little voice gets.

Don't Let Yourself Down

Here's what it comes down to. Anytime you listen to that little voice or are making an excuse, you're letting yourself down. It's time to stop doing that. Now is the time to honest with yourself. Realize what you're doing is sabotaging your success and Stop It! You're important and so is your health and well-being. If you haven't believed that yet, now is the time to start putting yourself first because no one else will.

Whenever you're tempted to skip a workout or indulge in an extra treat tell yourself that you won't let yourself down. Put on those walking shoes and head out for a workout. Make a smart choice about the food you eat. Skip the soda and reach for a bottle of water instead. Don't let yourself down.

You Are Worth It

You are worth the effort and hard work it is going to take to get down to a healthy weight. You are worth a healthy body that will support you in all endeavors for years and years to come.

We often focus on getting thin and more attractive for other people. Instead, do this for you because you know deep down that you are worth it. It's a much stronger motivator and no matter what happens with relationships along the way, your goal won't change.

You Deserve The Best

You deserve a long and happy life. You deserve being able to go to any store in the mall and find a cute outfit that fits. You deserve being able to go on that beautiful hike in the mountains. You deserve having a fun game of tag with the kids in the park. You deserve to be the person you already see inside yourself.

Stop making excuses and remember that you are worth it, you deserve the best and don't even think about letting yourself down.

Getting Back On Track – How To Pick Yourself Up After Falling Off Your Diet

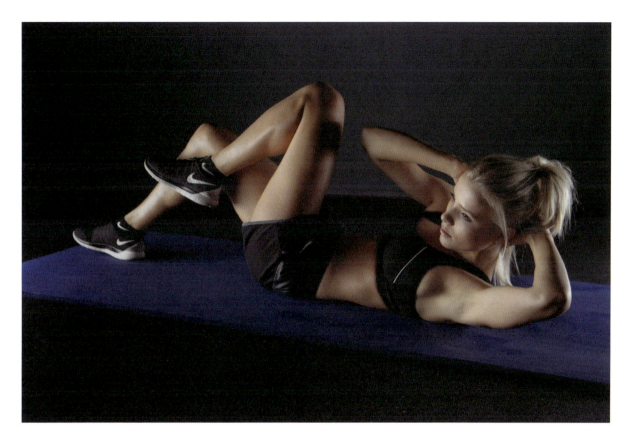

No matter how motivated and dedicated you are, chances are good that you'll fall off your diet at one point or another. It may be because you had a rough day at work and fell back into the old trap of making yourself feel better with food.

It could be that you were invited to a friend's house and she served some delicious homemade cake. Or maybe you "took a break" over the holidays to indulge a bit in all your favorite treats.

Perhaps you got sick and needed some comfort food to make you feel better. There are hundreds of reasons why we get off track of our goals. Let's accept that it's going to happen. No need to beat yourself up about it. What's important is what you do next.

How are you going to get back on track and keep this cheat meal or that indulgence day from turning into days and weeks of eating junk food, undoing all the hard work you've put in so far?

Forgive Yourself

First and foremost, there's no sense in beating yourself up. What's done is done. Forgive yourself and vow to do better in the future. Without forgiveness you'll beat yourself up for "failing" instead of just taking the next step forward. That's all you need to do to be successful. Just keep on moving forward!

Flush Out The "Bad" Stuff

Many convenience foods and sugar in particular can be quite addictive, making it hard to get back on track. I find it helps to eat exceptionally clean for at least a day and drink as much water and herbal tea as possible to flush out the "bad" stuff. It makes it easier to get right back on track and stick to your meal plans. Whole foods, homemade foods and things that come from nature are always better choices than anything from a box.

Recognize Triggers

After you've gotten back on track, take a look back and see if you can figure out why you slipped up. What caused you to reach for that tub of ice cream or why did you cave into eating that pizza after having the best intentions of sticking to a grilled chicken salad? Emotional triggers are huge saboteurs of an otherwise healthy eating plan.

Recognizing what's causing you to give in will help you avoid future slip ups.

Make A Plan To Avoid Future Slip Ups

Speaking of which, come up with some scenarios on what you can do next time to stay on plan.

For example, if you were meeting friends for dinner and ended up ordering the pizza or burger because you were just too hungry to consider getting the salad, have a snack before you leave the house.

If you're so busy that it was easier to pull through a fast-food drive through then think about planning ahead a little better.

If you had a bad day and found yourself reaching for the pint of Chunky Monkey in your freezer then consider not even bringing it into the house.

I hope these tips help you get back on track and reach your weight loss goals.

How To Set Smart Weight Loss Goals

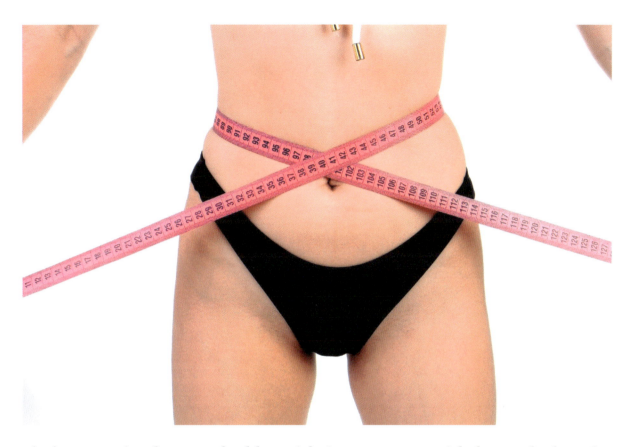

The key to getting down to a healthy weight is to set smart weight loss goals along the way. Let's talk about that for a minute. It's easy to come up with a number in your head and decide that you want to lose 15 pounds. You may even have an end date in mind. Maybe there's a wedding you're going to or you're headed off on a nice vacation in 2 months.

Having a specific goal and a deadline is a great start. Next you want to make sure it's a realistic goal. You want to be able to make it in the time allotted. It's good to make it a little ambitious but don't expect to lose more than a pound per week on average.

Speaking of weeks. It's good to have weekly and monthly goals. It'll help you notice the progress you're making and will keep you motivated. Once you have your smart weight loss goal set, it's time to get to work.

The fastest way to lose weight is a two-pronged approach. You want to change what you eat (and how much) and you want to move around more. Not only will you start to see the pounds melt off, but you'll also find yourself feeling better and with more energy.

As far as diet goes, we recommend eating clean, natural food. You want to cut out as much processed foods and sweets as possible. If you're looking for some good guidelines to follow, look into Whole 30. It's a 30-Day Clean Eating Challenge that will get you on the right track when it comes to food and drink.

When it comes to exercise pick something that's fun and that you're comfortable with. Just about anyone can go out for a walk. Pick up a pedometer like a FitBit, lace up your walking shoes and go out there. Set a daily stepping goal. You may want to start out walking 7,000 steps per day and then increase that number by another 1,000 steps every few weeks.

Make a goal of moving at least 1 hour per day but remember you can break that down into 15-minute increments, too. 15 minutes in the morning right after you wake up – set your alarm clock early if you need to. Another 15 minutes before lunch, 15 more after lunch and 15 after dinner will have your daily requirements met easy peasy.

Last but not least, weight loss is about more than just the number on the scale. Take a few other measurements including body fat percentage and take out a measuring tape and take your chest, waist, thigh and upper arm measurements. Write those numbers down. Often you'll lose inches even if the scale insists on giving you the same number day after day.

While the scale might not be moving as quickly as you want it to, take stock of those other measurements as well as how you feel physically and emotionally. Finally, how are those clothes fitting? A little looser than they used to, I'd bet.

Set Yourself Up For Success – How To Stick To Your Weight Loss Goals

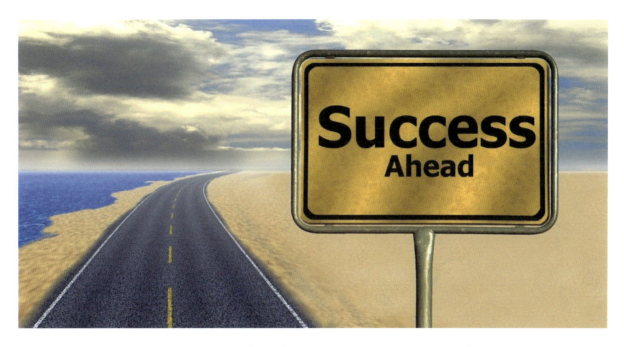

Setting weight loss goals is great, but the hard part is sticking to the plan and reaching your final goal. Today I want to share 8 tips with you that will set you up for success. Ready to learn how to stick to your weight loss goals? Here we go.

Use Visualization

Visualization is a powerful tool. Close your eyes and picture yourself at your ideal weight. How do you look? How does it feel? How will you feel being able to run around the park with the kids or climbing up those stairs without running out of breath? Paint a clear picture in your mind of the lean you. Make it a habit to visualize this slim and healthy version of yourself daily.

Create Accountability

Sometimes it's just a little too easy to make bad choices. That chocolate cookie won't hurt, and it's not that big of a deal to skip a workout. Before you know it that whole plate of cookies is gone, and you haven't been out to walk for over a week. Accountability will help you keep on track. Find a friend who also wants to lose weight and hold each other accountable. Or ask a loved one to keep you straight.

If this sounds a little too intimidating or just isn't your thing, consider keeping a journal. Just knowing that you'll have to write down that piece of cheesecake is enough motivation to pick an apple instead.

Make It Attainable

You want to push yourself, but you also want to make sure they are actually reachable. Setting a huge goal like losing 30 pounds can seem almost insurmountable. Instead, start with a smaller goal like losing 10 pounds over the next 2 months. Then set another 10-pound goal and repeat until you reach your weight goal.

Take Breaks

If you have attainable goals and some accountability in place, it's ok to take a little break every once in a while. Take a break from your workout. In fact, except for low impact exercise like going for a walk, you don't want to overdo it. 3 to 5 days at the gym is plenty. And it's ok to have a piece of birthday cake on occasion. Just make sure you work on getting exercise and eating healthy 90% of the time.

Create Good Habits

Which brings us to another great tip. Use this time to work on creating healthy habits. Make going for that daily walk part of your new lifestyle. Make eating three healthy meals a family habit. Not only will it set you up for success now, but those healthy habits will also help you keep the weight off long after you've reached your goal.

Celebrate

Losing weight is hard work. Don't forget to celebrate each success. If you made it out for a 30 minute walk each day this week, celebrate with a mini movie marathon. Did you lose your first 15 pounds? Take yourself out to get your nails done or treat yourself to a cute new top. Reward yourself for each success and milestone reached.

Lifestyle Changes

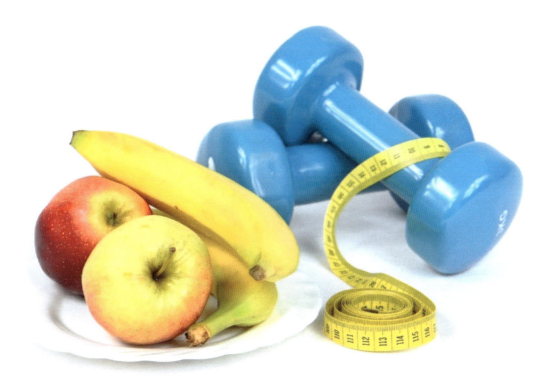

#1 - Eat Less

Let's start with the hardest habit to get into. It's to eat less. It makes sense, doesn't it? You eat less, you'll start to lose weight. Or at least you'll stop gaining pounds.

Over the past few decades our portions have gotten bigger and bigger. We're bad about piling food on our large plates (yes, our plates have gotten bigger too) and then finishing it all no matter what.

Instead, let's get in the habit of eating a little less, eating a little slower and stopping when we start to get full. Here are some simple little hacks to help us do that.

Portion Control

Our portions have gotten bigger and bigger. And we're used to eating long past the point where we start to feel full. It's time to retrain ourselves to get a feel for how much a serving of pasta, chicken, rice, corn, cereal or anything else on our plate should be.

Start by reading up on portions and invest in an inexpensive set of measuring cups. You can even use your hand in a pinch. Here are some general guidelines:

- 1 cup = your fist
- 1 ounce = the meaty part of your thumb
- 1 tablespoon = your thumb, minus the meaty part
- 1 teaspoon = the tip of your index finger
- 1 inch = the middle section of your index finger
- 1-2 ounces of a food like nuts or pretzels = your cupped hand
- 3 ounces of meat, fish, or poultry = the palm of your hand

Measure your food for a few days until you have a feel for what you should be eating.

Getting out a smaller plate or bowl will also help you dish out smaller portions.

Once you have your plate, fill it up with leafy greens, vegetables and a little fruit first. Add a portion of meat and only then add the rest. The idea is that you'll have less room for the stuff that's bad for you.

Group Your Foods Correctly

Last but not least try to group your foods together so they don't make your blood sugar spike. Blood sugar spikes are what make use crave even more food a little later. Don't eat carbs and particularly sugary foods by themselves. Instead combine them with a protein or even a little healthy fat. It'll keep your blood sugar levels more even and avoid insulin spikes.

It also helps to eat a serving of leafy greens anytime you have a meal or snack. These low calorie veggies are good for you and will fill you up without adding a lot of calories.

Drink Plenty Of Water

Last but not least make sure you drink plenty of water. Having a big glass of water with dinner will help fill you up quicker.

But there's more to it than just helping with portion control. We often confuse thirst and hunger (or those cravings). If in doubt, have some water and see if you were "just" thirsty.

#2 - Eat Better

We already touched on this but getting healthy is all about eating food that's better for you. Skip the cookies, chips and donuts and fill up with food that nourishes your body. Yes, it's tough in the beginning, particularly because refined carbs and sugar are addictive compounds, but it will get easier.

It'll well be worth it when you start to have more energy, feel better and realize that real food actually tastes much better than the factory made stuff.

Less Sugar

Start by cutting out the sugar. If you can make do without oversweet coffee drinks and breakfast cereals loaded with sugar, you'll be amazed at how much clearer your head will be. And you won't have that mid-morning slump either.

Pay attention to labels and cut sugar anywhere you can. Cook from scratch when possible and choose non-sugary foods whenever possible. Stop eating cereal or pop tarts for breakfast and scramble up some eggs instead.

If you're craving a little something sweet, pick some fruit instead of heading for the candy bowl. Frozen grapes make a yummy sweet treat. Or freeze some banana slices and either dip them in melted chocolate for a candy-bar like treat or blend them up with some milk for mock ice cream.

Less Carbs

Eating less sugar will cut out quite a few carbs from your diet, but don't just stop there. Cut back on white foods like bread, pasta, rice, potatoes and the likes.

Reading labels and learning a little bit about nutrition is important here. IT's amazing how often carbs are snuck into all sorts of foods we eat each day.

Wheat has gotten a bad rep over the past few years and even if you aren't gluten intolerant, it's a good idea to cut as much wheat out of your diet as possible.

Don't forget about drinks either. Fruit juices and sodas are full of sugar (which is a carb) and let's not even get stared with beer. Yes, the occasional treat is fine, but overall aim to eat less carbohydrates.

More Protein

So what do you eat instead? Cutting down on carbs limits a whole bunch of food we typically eat. We'll talk about vegetables in a minute, but first let's talk about protein. It takes much longer to digest protein than it does carbs. Protein will keep you full longer. In other words, you won't get hungry two hours after you eat.

Protein is also great at mellowing out any potential insulin spikes carbs can cause. Try to eat at least a small portion of protein with each meal.

There's a reason why we need at least a little protein each day. It contains building blocks (amino acids) our bodies need to keep regenerating.

Protein is found in meat but also in vegetables particularly legumes (think beans).

More Non-Starchy Veggies

I already mentioned that a good trick to make yourself eat healthier is to fill up on leafy green vegetable. Really any non-starchy veggie is a good choice. Not only do they fill you up without a lot of calories, they are also full of vitamins and other micro-nutrients that are important for a healthy body.

When I mention leafy green vegetables, you're probably thinking salad. Salads are great, but don't just stop there. Make a pot of vegetable soup, stew up some cabbage or collard greens, and cook up a pot of spinach. Or add your veggies to a smoothie. There are some great green smoothie recipes out there. Try blending up banana, romaine lettuce and water into a yummy sweet green smoothies. Or blend up spinach, coconut water and frozen blueberries. Play around with green smoothie recipes. Just try to stay away from adding fruit juices. We don't want to turn our healthy smoothie into a sugary treat.

Healthy Fats

Let's talk about fat for a minute. Low fat didn't work. We did it since the early 70s, cutting out each and every little bit of fat from our diet. And we've gotten fatter and fatter in the process. We need fat to keep running, keep our energy up and keep us full longer.

But fat isn't just fat. Skip the margarine and use some grass fed butter instead. Stock up on nuts, seeds and avocados.

A word of caution. While some fat is good for us, it can also pack on calories that we may not need. Incorporate healthy fats into your diet daily, but be sure to pay attention to portion size when you do.

#3 - Move More

To stay healthy we have to move around more. Most of us have very sedentary lives. We sit at a desk and when we get home, we sit back down in front of the TV.

But exercising is hard. We start the New Year with the best of intentions and even sign up for a gym membership. We do well for a week or two and then slip back into bad habits. We make excuses why we can't go exercise.

So don't think about it as exercising. Just tell yourself you are going to move around more. And it doesn't have these long marathon sessions. Start with 15 minutes. Even 15 minutes more than you're moving now helps and those 15 minutes will start to add up.

Take a little walk on your lunch break or after dinner. Dance around the living room with your kids or go play around at the park. Make it fun and keep it easy. Just remind yourself several times a day to move more.

#4 - Choose Your Passion

Find something that gets you moving without you even realizing you're "exercising". Have you ridden a bike in a while? It's a lot of fun. Or sign up for some dance lessons. Think about anything active you've enjoyed in the past and rediscover your passion.

And don't be afraid to try something new. You never know what may be fun. Go out and try things like tennis, mini golf and pickle ball. Go walk on the beach and look for shells or go on a nature walk.

Sign up for a kayaking tour or take up fishing. Plant a garden, go for a swim. The sky is the limit. Find something you enjoy that gets you moving. If it gets you moving outside, that's even better.

And let's not forget people. People make an experience even more fun. Join a walking group or get some friends together to play basketball at the local rec center. Or join a yoga class and see if you don't make some new friends.

#5 - Get Support

Since we're talking about people, let's keep going and talk about support. Our support system is what will keep us going when we feel like giving up. They keep us motivated and push us to do even better.

Find a group of like-minded people, preferably with the same lifestyle change goals, to help keep you accountable.

Find supporters who will encourage you to keep on moving even after you've eaten an entire box of doughnuts (the whole dozen). Let's be real... it's going to happen. We all slip up, make bad choices and fall back into bad habits.

That's why having a strong support system in place is so important. This can be people who eat what you eat, want to lose the same amount of weight you do, and go exercising with you. It can be, but it doesn't have to be. They can also be loved ones, family and friends who are there to cheer you on and keep you accountable.

Don't limit yourself to just local people. You can build an amazing team of supporters online as well. Join some groups and forums to connect with other people on a journey similar to yours. Find your tribe and communicate with them daily. Cheer each other on and call each other out when someone hasn't check in or slipped up.

It's not easy getting healthy, but I hope this short report has given you some ideas to get started on the journey to a healthier and happier you.

Smart Apps To Help You Reach Your Weight Loss Goals

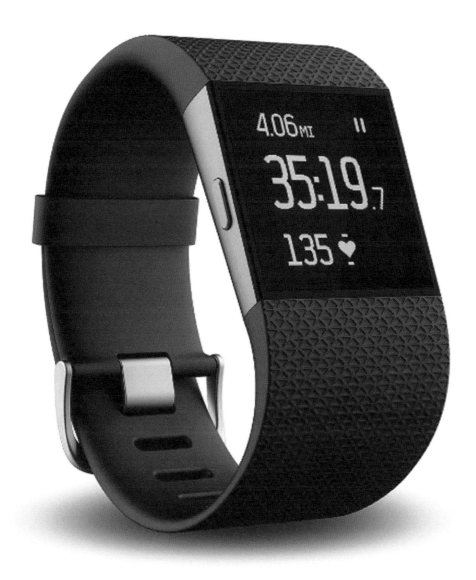

I love my smart phone. It's such an amazing little device and there really is an app for just about anything. And there are plenty of smart apps that can help you reach your weight loss goal. Here are five of my favorites. Check them out and see if they can't help you eat better, move more and melt off those extra pounds.

My Fitness Pal

My Fitness Pal is a website, online community and mobile app that allows you to track your food, calories, workouts, and weight. I love how easily the app integrates with the website. It makes it easy to use your computer to do anything that involves a lot of typing (for example when you first start to enter and track the food you typically eat).

Then you can use the app to continue tracking on the go and check your stats. The online community has a wealth of information and support built in. There is a huge database of foods for you to work with and it's free for both iPhone and android devices.

FitBit

The FitBit app itself is free, but only works with a Fitbit device. A fitbit is a pedometer or step counter on steroids, giving you all sorts of great data. Find out how many steps you walk, how many flights of stairs you climb and even how well you sleep at night. It's a nice motivational tool to get you moving more.

Much like My Fitness Pal it also lets you track your food and other exercise. You can also track your weight and compete with other fitbit users to see how much you can walk in a day.

My personal favorite is the little badges you get (via email) for various different accomplishments like reaching your daily goals and all-time steps walked. It's very motivating and keeps me going.

Pedometer And Weight Loss Coach

This app uses your phone's built-in pedometer to do what a Fitbit device does. This works great if you have you phone on you most of the day.

The app interface is very simple and easy to use. Set some goals, start tracking how much you move and keep going. Walking is one of the easiest exercises to do and it's quite effective in getting you slimmed down and healthy.

Ideal Weight

Knowing your BMI is good way to know where you're at with your weight and where you should be. But calculating Body Mass Index by hand can be a little daunting.

The ideal weight app makes it easy to get an accurate calculation. You can also play around and see how many pounds you need to lose to get your BMI number to move down. It's a nice tool to have to set milestones along your weight loss journey.

Noom Coach

This is another app that allows you to track your food and how much you walk in a given day. What I love about this particular app is that it focuses on making new healthy habits instead of "going on a diet".

This is by no means an all-inclusive list. There are plenty of other good apps out there. I chose the ones above because they are available for both iPhone and android devices.

Tools To Help You Reach Your Weight Loss Goals

```
Day: S / M / T / W / Th / F / S    Date: _____

Goals / Inspiration For Today:



Water: ☐☐☐☐☐☐        Fruit / Veggies: ☐☐☐☐☐☐
```

BREAKFAST	CALORIES	SNACKS	CALORIES

LUNCH	CALORIES	EXERCISE

DINNER	CALORIES	Thoughts & Reflections

Losing weight is hard work and we can all use a little extra help. Here are four different things you may want to have in your tool belt. They'll help keep you on track and more importantly keep you motivated to keep going. Motivation is key, particularly on those days when you're craving high calorie food or don't want to head outside to exercise. Use these tools to help you reach your weight loss goals.

Food and Exercise Journal

One of the simplest, yet most effective tools to accompany on your weight loss journey is a journal. Use it to record what you're eating when, how much water you're drinking and what exercises you're doing in a given day. You might be surprised with what you find out.

You may also want to record how you're feeling on any given day and what challenges you've encountered during the day. Just knowing that you'll have to write it down is often enough motivation to keep you from overeating and to head out for a walk.

A Vision Board

The mind is a powerful thing and it can be a strong ally to you. Spend a little time each day picturing the thinner, healthier version of you that you're destined to become. A vision board can be helpful here. Get a piece of construction paper and add anything that helps you visualize the thinner you.

Use pictures of yourself when you were down to your ideal weight. Or find magazine pictures of people that looks similar to you and are the shape you want to get down to. You can also add images of the types of outfits you plan on wearing after your weight loss, and of course plenty of pictures describing the lifestyle and activities you look forward to.

An Outfit In Your Ideal Size

Is there a particular outfit you look forward to wearing? Or is there a jeans size you are trying to get down to? Go ahead and buy a pair and hang it up in your bedroom. Look at it each day and tell yourself that you're well on your way to fitting those pants.

You may also want to keep one pair of pants from your heaviest days. When you feel like you're not making progress, pull them on as a strong visual reminder of how far you've come. This will be very powerful as soon as you start losing inches around your waist (which will happen quickly).

A Support Group

Last but not least let's talk about support from others. Surround yourself with people that support and encourage your weight loss journey. Ask them to hold you accountable and cheer you on.

This support group can happen locally with loved ones and friends, but it can also be an online group. It's even more powerful when you can find others who are working hard to lose pounds and get in shape. You can cheer each other on and help each other along your weight loss journey.

From Overweight to In Shape - 6 Smart Goal Setting Tips

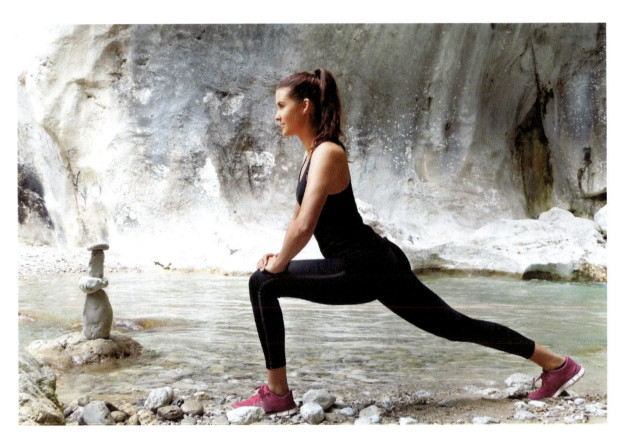

Losing weight isn't easy. The truth is that no matter what the advertising for the latest and greatest diet product promises, it's hard work. And it'll take you a while. That sounds pretty discouraging, doesn't it? I'm here to offer some help. The single most effective "tool" I've found for sustainable weight loss is to set smart weight loss goals. What makes a goal smart? Read on to find out.

Find Your Focus

Losing weight won't happen overnight. What will make it happen is developing better eating habits and moving more. Those are lifestyle changes, and it will take a while before they become habits for you. In the meantime, you will need to focus on practicing your new habits daily while focusing on your goal at the same time. If you have a concrete reason of why you want to lose weight you'll find that focus easier. Here are a few questions to ask yourself. Do I want to live a long, healthy life? Do I want to set a good example for my kids? Will I have a better quality of life if I make these changes? Find your focus and use it to reach your goals before this new lean lifestyle becomes a habit.

Be Specific

Saying "I need to lose some weight" just doesn't cut it. Sorry to be so harsh, but it's the truth. You need to be more specific. Set a weight loss goal. Pick a number. How many pounds do you want to lose? How many inches do you want to whittle from your waist? Be specific. The only way you'll know when you've reached your goal is to have a number in mind to reach. Otherwise, while you might make progress, you'll never reach your goal.

Set Yourself A Deadline

Someone smart once told me that goals without deadlines are just dreams. There's a lot of truth in that statement. Without a deadline, you have no frame of reference. As specific as wanting to lose 25 pounds is, without a deadline it could take you a year or a decade. Smart goals have a realistic deadline. Losing a pound per week is an ambitious but realistic goal. Losing 25 pounds in the next 6 months is a smart goal with a deadline.

Celebrate Your Victories

Changing your eating habits and getting your body moving isn't easy, especially if you've been a couch potato until now. Stay motivated by breaking your big goal into little mini goals and celebrating your victories along the way. If your end goal is to lose 25 pounds in 6 months, break it down into 5-pound increments. Give yourself a pat on the back and do something nice or fun to celebrate each 5-pound loss. Just try not to use food as a reward.

Get Real

Don't set your goals so high you'll get discouraged when you don't meet them. Losing 100 pounds in 3 months just isn't going to happen. You don't want to set yourself up for failure. Instead, set yourself up for success with goals that you can reach … but don't be afraid to have to stretch a bit to reach them.

And don't get discouraged if you fall of the wagon every now and again. Life happens and sometimes there's just no way to say no to that slice of pizza (or two, or three). The important thing is to pick yourself right back up and keep working towards your goals.

Stay Accountable

It's nice to have someone that has your back. Find an accountability partner. Ideally this person will be on a weight loss journey as well. You can support and encourage each other. You can call each other out when you're binging on junk food or skipping your walk yet again. Share your goals with your accountability partner and have him or her hold you to them.

Now it's your turn. Ready to set some smart weight loss goals?

Reaching Weight Loss Milestones - Don't Forget To Celebrate Your Success

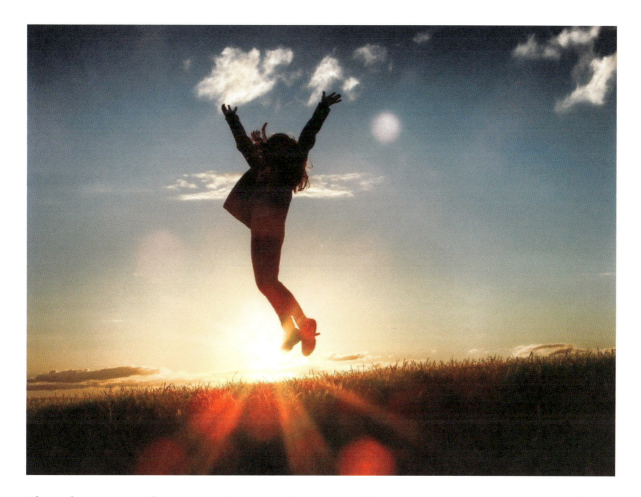

If you have more than just a few pounds to lose, it's not going to happen overnight. It took a while to put on the extra weight, so it shouldn't come as a huge surprise that it will also take some time to take it back off. But that can seem a bit discouraging at times. One way to stay motivated is to set different little mini goals or weight loss milestones. Don't forget that each time you reach a milestone you should celebrate your success and how far you've come on your weight loss journey.

When you set your milestones is entirely up to you. It partially depends on how much weight you have to lose. If you're motivated by rewards, you may want to set plenty of little milestones along the way. It's easier to make and meet smaller goals – like 1-3 lbs. The more realistic the goal the easier they are to reach, too.

Each pound lost is a success. Celebrating after every 5 pounds might be a good starting point.

It's a big enough goal that you have to really try to get there, but it won't take you ages. You don't want to have too much time between milestones, so you don't lose steam along the way.

I recommend you don't use food as a reward. You don't want to reinforce bad eating habits by using food as a reward. Instead, thing of other fun things. Get a new book, buy a new outfit, get a massage or buy some new makeup. Mani/pedi anyone? Even simple things like taking some time to just curl up on the couch with a cup of tea watching a movie can be a nice reward. Pick something that you want and that makes you work for that next weight loss milestone.

Another fun option is to make a poster similar to the ones used at fundraisers. Mark down each pound you lose and have it hanging up in your bedroom or bathroom. It will be a nice visual reminder of how well you're doing and how much weight you've lost already.

Recording milestones and celebrating each one is a powerful motivator. Don't be shy about sharing your success with others. Having your loved ones celebrate with you and cheer you on can be very helpful. Making your weight loss journey "public knowledge" also helps to hold you accountable. You'll be even more motivated to keep going and stick with the program if you have to admit to your family that you're giving up.

Keep going, stay motivated, set some milestones and celebrate your success.

About the Author

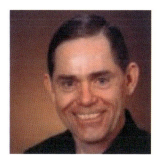

 I am a published writer with numerous books on Amazon for Kindle and other publishing platforms ... both in electronic and Print On Demand (POD) formats.

While most of my self-published books are on health and fitness in general, my topics of interest currently are more toward 1) aging baby boomers and the older population and 2) low content books, like word activity books, journals, planners and calendars.

Besides my own writing, I also ghostwrite ebooks, books, reports, articles, autoresponder series, blogs and Kindle conversions for my client base on a variety of topics. I'm currently using Microsoft's Office Suite including Word, Powerpoint and Publisher, along with Affinity Publisher and Designrr for writing and publishing.

Go to my website at http://ronknesswriting.com for more information or to request a quote: https://ronknesswriting.com/ghostwriting-quote-request-form.

For a complete list of my books published on Amazon, go to https://www.amazon.com/Ron-Kness/e/B0072M6PYO.

Today my wife and I are retired from our careers and live in Queen Creek, AZ. I now write as a retirement business where you'll find me happily sitting in my office typing away on my computer as I work on my next book or ghostwriting project for a client . . . that is if we are not traveling somewhere in our RV - our renewed mode of travel.

Take care and be safe!

Ron

Printed in Great Britain
by Amazon